# THIS PLANNER
# BELONGS TO

0 0 0 0 0 0 0 0 0 0 0 0 0 0 0 0 0 0 0 0 0 0 0 0 0 0 0 0 0 0 0 0 0

# Index

Introduction

Date

No of attendees

Warm up

Private Class

Main body

Notes

Feedback

Cool down

☆☆☆☆☆

## Introduction

## Date

## Warm up

## No of attendees

## Private Class

## Notes

## Main body

## Feedback

## Cool down

☆☆☆☆☆

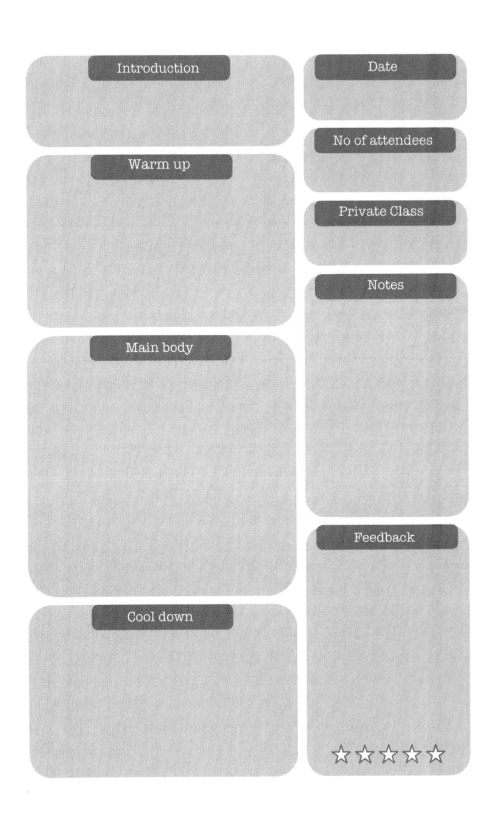

Introduction

Date

Warm up

No of attendees

Private Class

Main body

Notes

Feedback

Cool down

☆☆☆☆☆

## Introduction

## Warm up

## Main body

## Cool down

## Date

## No of attendees

## Private Class

## Notes

## Feedback

☆ ☆ ☆ ☆ ☆

## Introduction

## Date

## Warm up

## No of attendees

## Private Class

## Main body

## Notes

## Cool down

## Feedback

☆☆☆☆☆

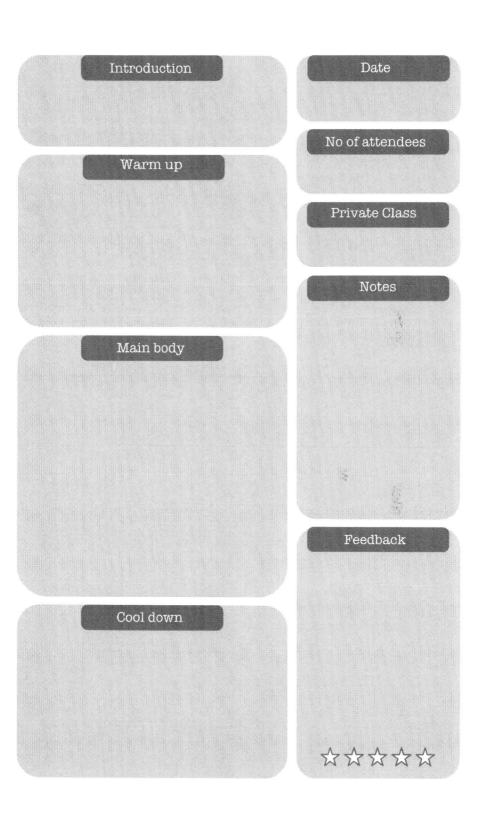

Introduction

Date

Warm up

No of attendees

Private Class

Main body

Notes

Feedback

Cool down

☆☆☆☆☆

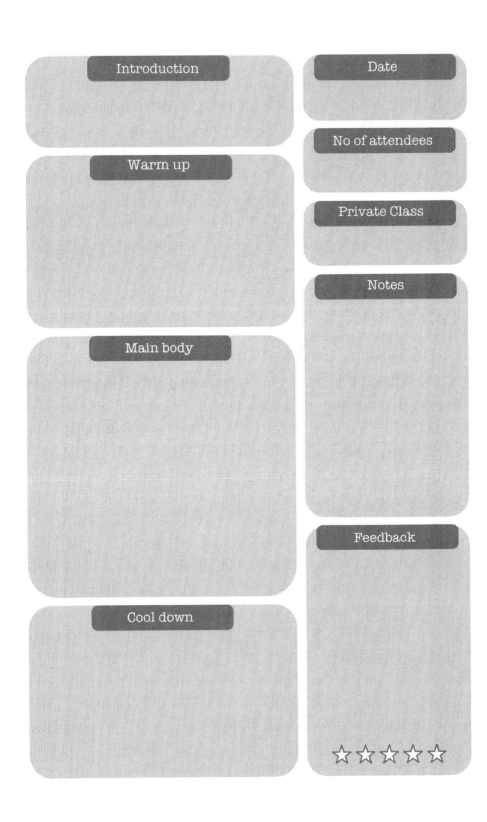

Introduction

Date

Warm up

No of attendees

Private Class

Main body

Notes

Cool down

Feedback

☆☆☆☆☆

## Introduction

## Date

## Warm up

## No of attendees

## Private Class

## Main body

## Notes

## Cool down

## Feedback

☆ ☆ ☆ ☆ ☆

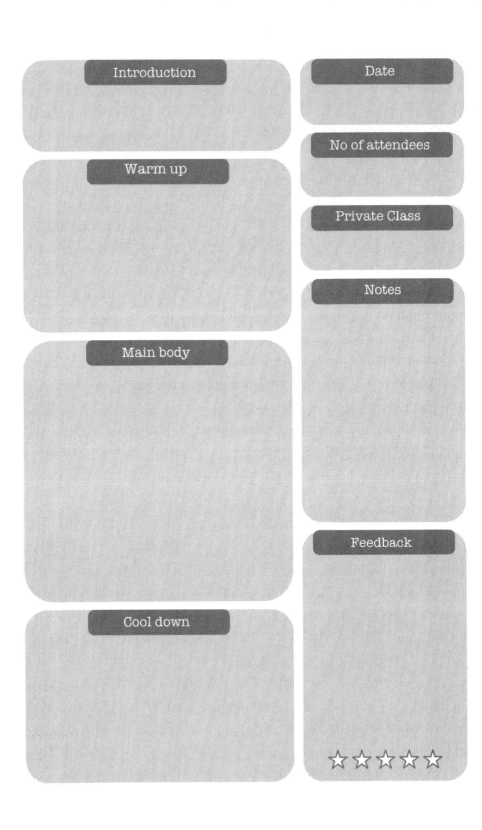

Introduction

Date

Warm up

No of attendees

Private Class

Main body

Notes

Feedback

Cool down

☆☆☆☆☆

## Introduction

## Warm up

## Main body

## Cool down

## Date

## No of attendees

## Private Class

## Notes

## Feedback

☆ ☆ ☆ ☆ ☆

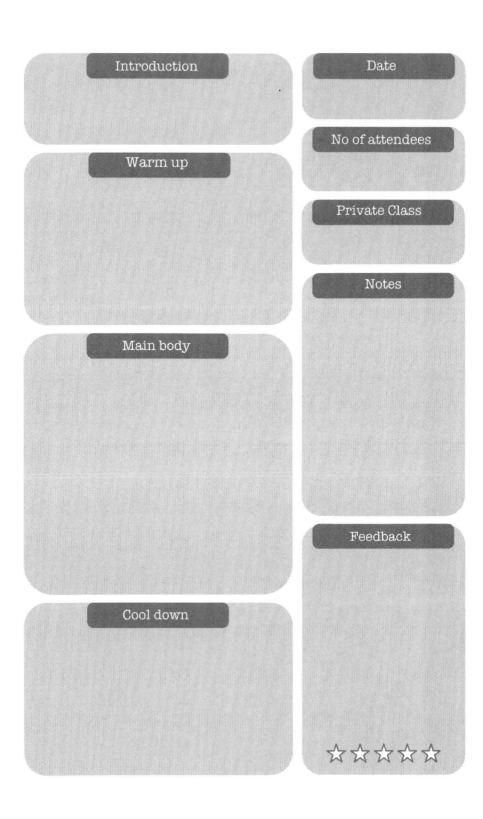

Introduction

Date

Warm up

No of attendees

Private Class

Main body

Notes

Cool down

Feedback

☆☆☆☆☆

## Introduction

## Date

## Warm up

## No of attendees

## Private Class

## Main body

## Notes

## Cool down

## Feedback

☆☆☆☆☆

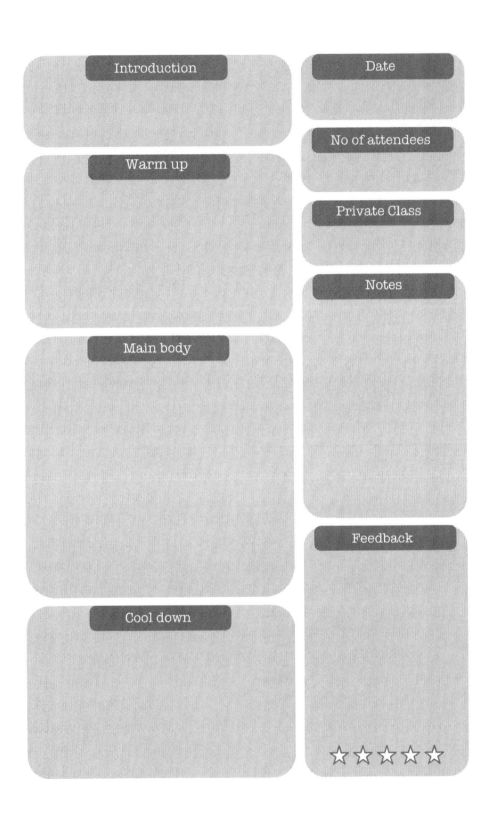

**Introduction**

**Date**

**Warm up**

**No of attendees**

**Private Class**

**Notes**

**Main body**

**Feedback**

**Cool down**

☆☆☆☆☆

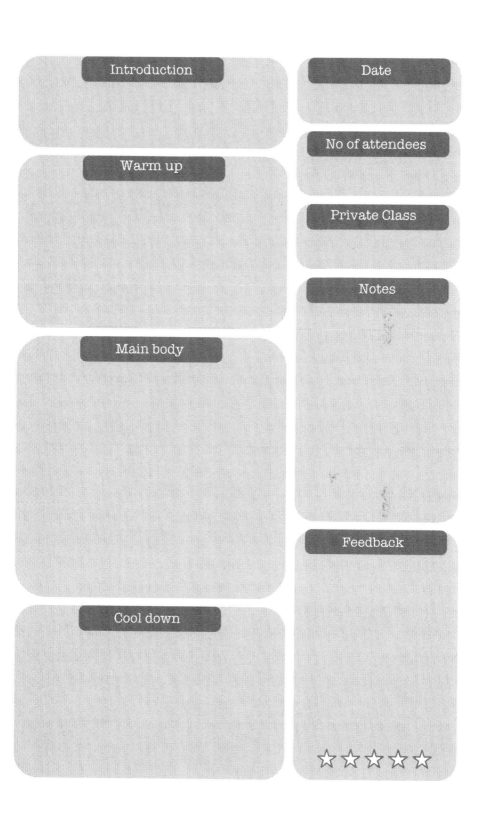

Introduction

Date

Warm up

No of attendees

Private Class

Main body

Notes

Cool down

Feedback

☆☆☆☆☆

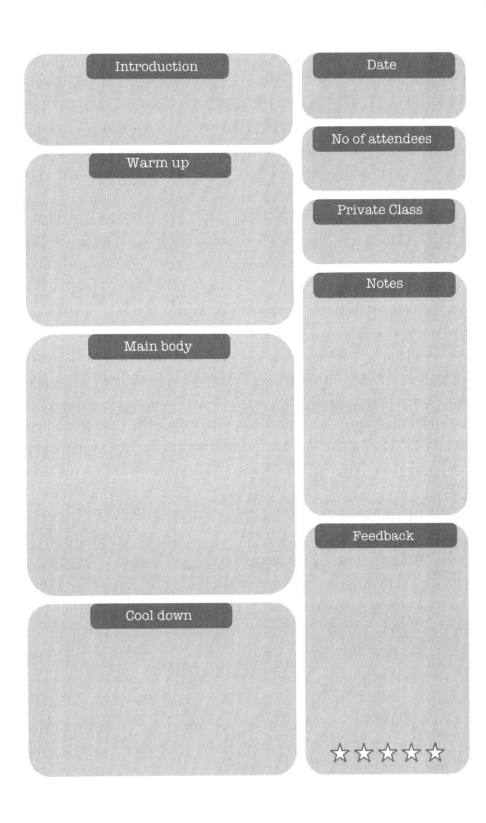

Introduction

Date

Warm up

No of attendees

Private Class

Main body

Notes

Feedback

Cool down

☆☆☆☆☆

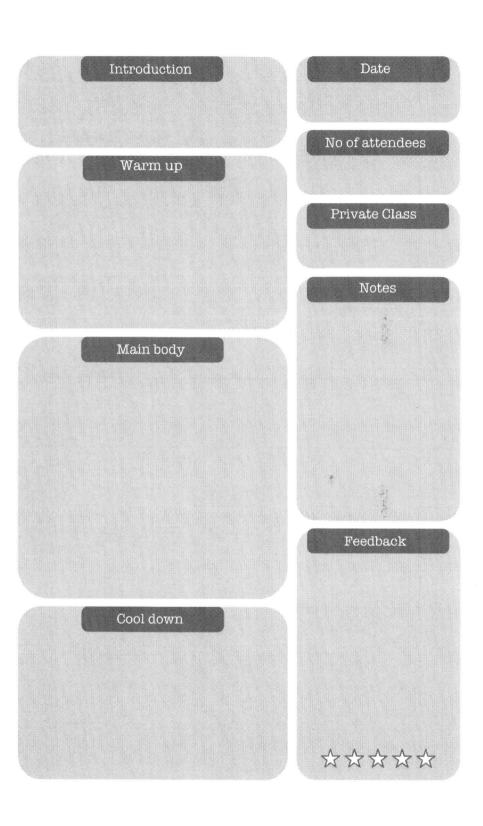

Introduction

Date

Warm up

No of attendees

Private Class

Main body

Notes

Feedback

Cool down

☆☆☆☆☆

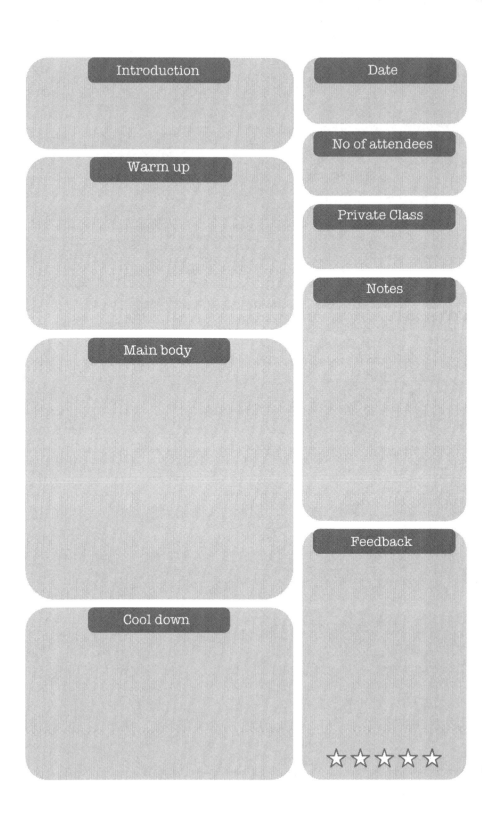

Introduction

Date

Warm up

No of attendees

Private Class

Main body

Notes

Feedback

Cool down

☆☆☆☆☆

## Introduction

## Warm up

## Main body

## Cool down

## Date

## No of attendees

## Private Class

## Notes

## Feedback

☆☆☆☆☆

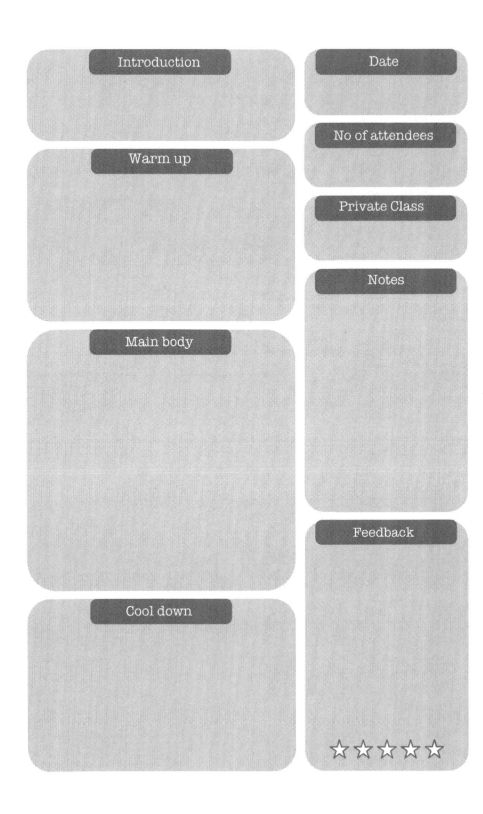

Introduction

Date

Warm up

No of attendees

Private Class

Main body

Notes

Feedback

Cool down

☆☆☆☆☆

## Introduction

## Date

## Warm up

## No of attendees

## Private Class

## Main body

## Notes

## Cool down

## Feedback

☆☆☆☆☆

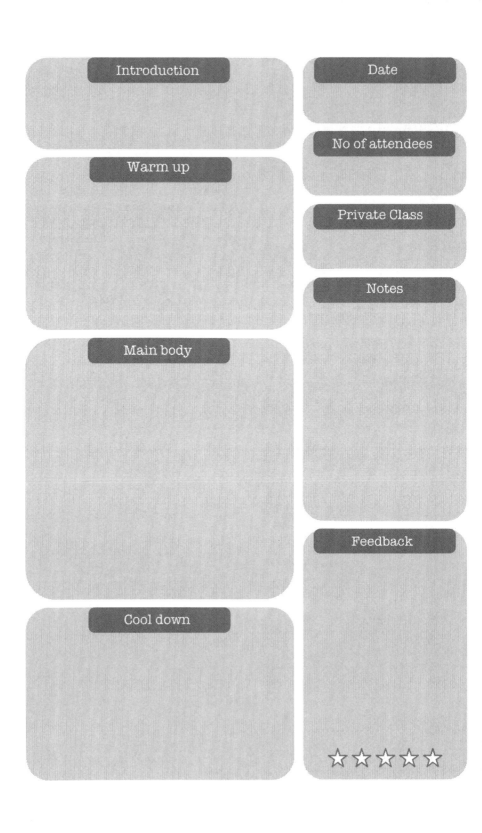

**Introduction**

**Date**

**Warm up**

**No of attendees**

**Private Class**

**Main body**

**Notes**

**Feedback**

**Cool down**

☆☆☆☆☆

## Introduction

## Date

## Warm up

## No of attendees

## Private Class

## Main body

## Notes

## Cool down

## Feedback

☆ ☆ ☆ ☆ ☆

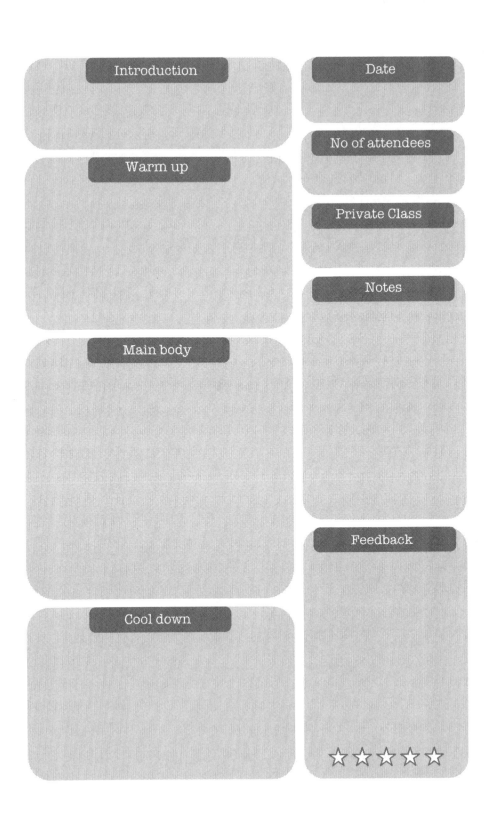

**Introduction**

**Date**

**No of attendees**

**Warm up**

**Private Class**

**Main body**

**Notes**

**Feedback**

**Cool down**

☆☆☆☆☆

## Introduction

## Date

## Warm up

## No of attendees

## Private Class

## Notes

## Main body

## Feedback

## Cool down

☆☆☆☆☆

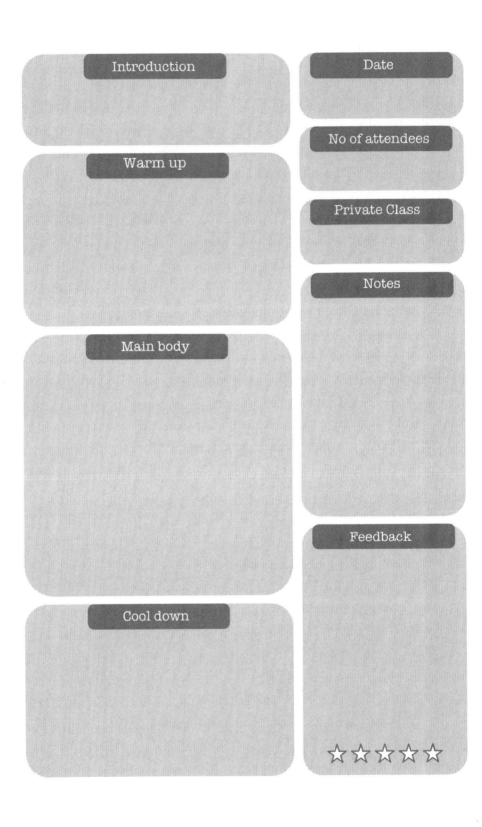

Introduction

Date

Warm up

No of attendees

Private Class

Main body

Notes

Feedback

Cool down

☆ ☆ ☆ ☆ ☆

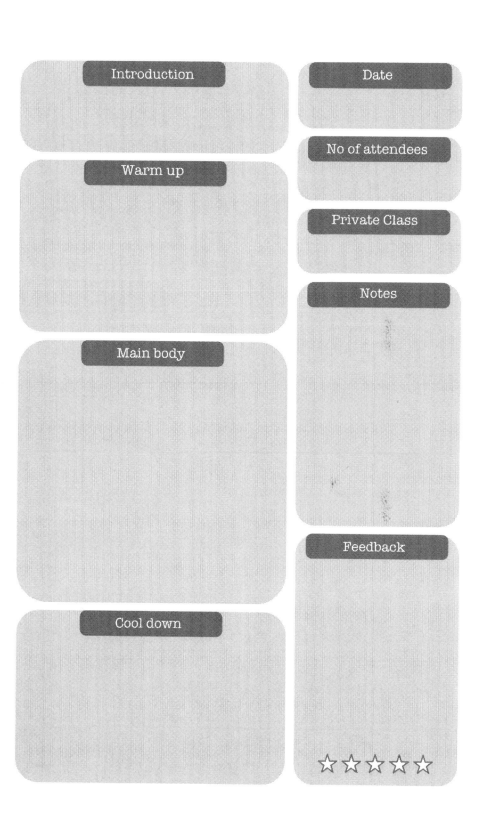

## Introduction

## Warm up

## Main body

## Cool down

## Date

## No of attendees

## Private Class

## Notes

## Feedback

☆☆☆☆☆

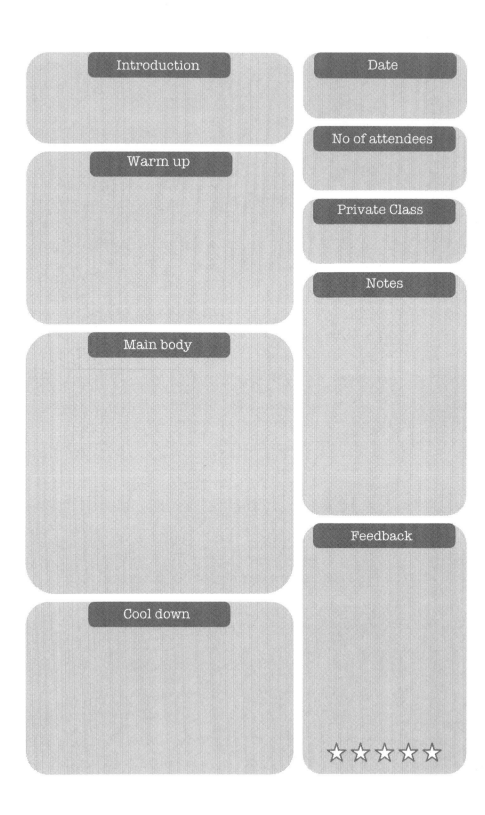

Introduction

Date

Warm up

No of attendees

Private Class

Main body

Notes

Feedback

Cool down

☆☆☆☆☆

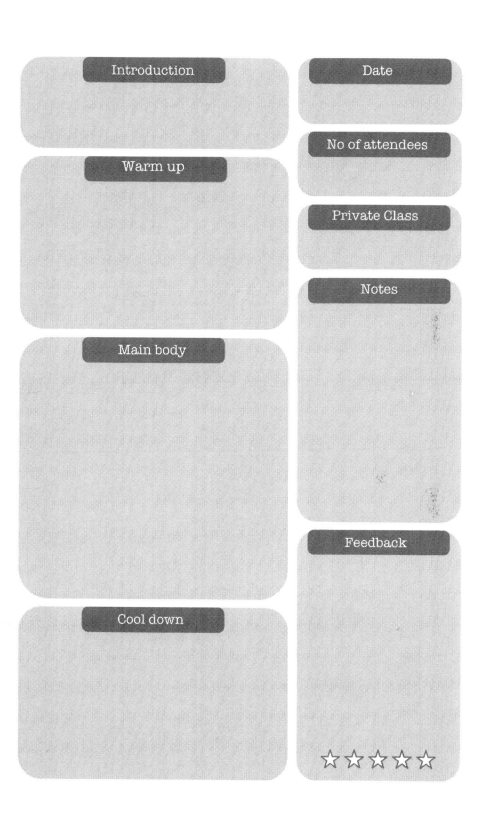

## Introduction

## Date

## Warm up

## No of attendees

## Private Class

## Notes

## Main body

## Cool down

## Feedback

☆ ☆ ☆ ☆ ☆

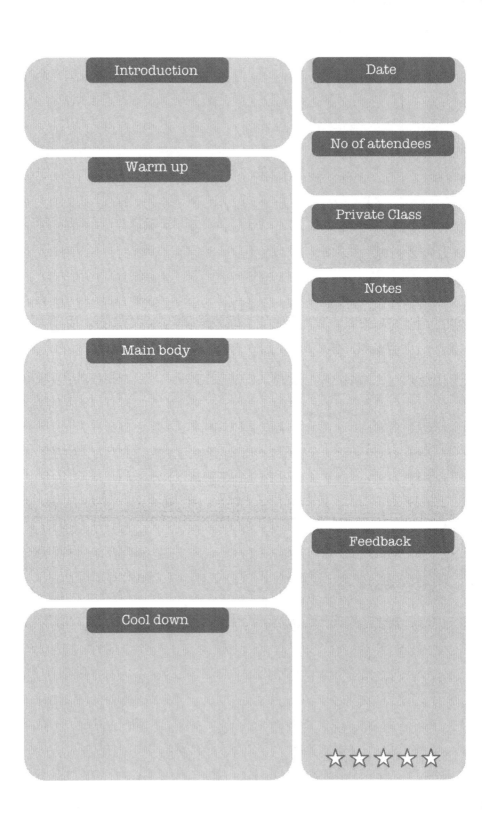

Introduction

Date

Warm up

No of attendees

Private Class

Main body

Notes

Feedback

Cool down

☆☆☆☆☆

## Introduction

## Warm up

## Main body

## Cool down

## Date

## No of attendees

## Private Class

## Notes

## Feedback

☆☆☆☆☆

## Introduction

## Warm up

## Main body

## Cool down

## Date

## No of attendees

## Private Class

## Notes

## Feedback

☆ ☆ ☆ ☆ ☆

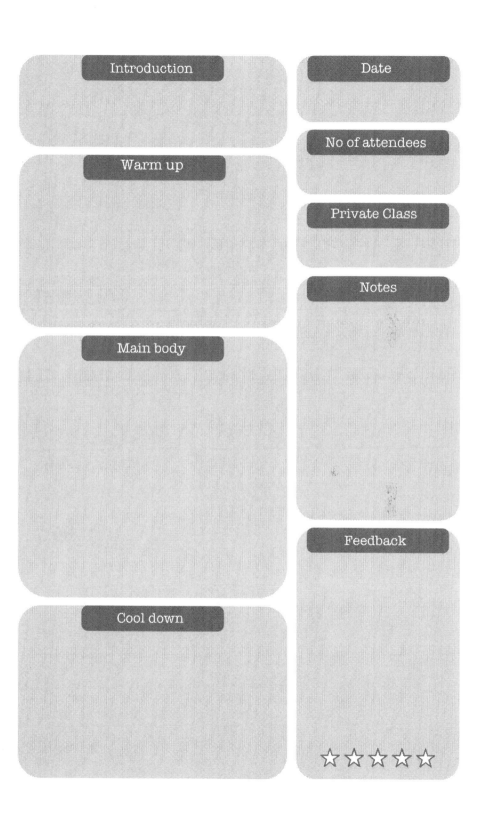

Introduction

Date

Warm up

No of attendees

Private Class

Main body

Notes

Cool down

Feedback

☆☆☆☆☆

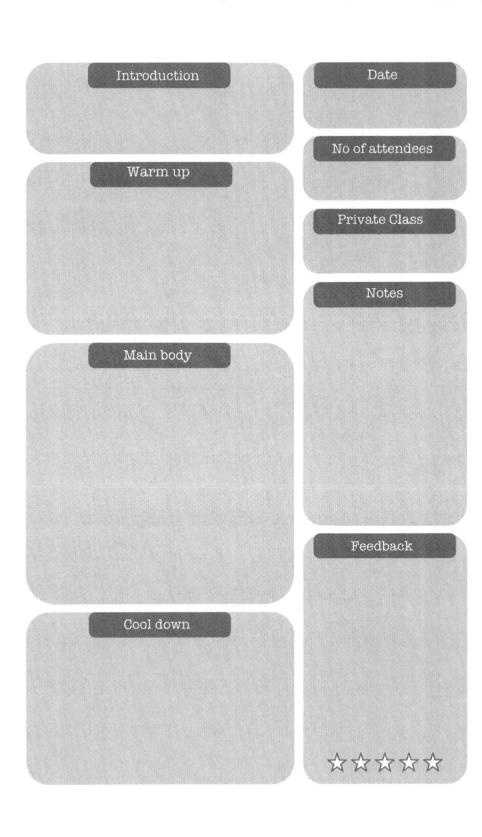

Introduction

Date

Warm up

No of attendees

Private Class

Main body

Notes

Feedback

Cool down

☆☆☆☆☆

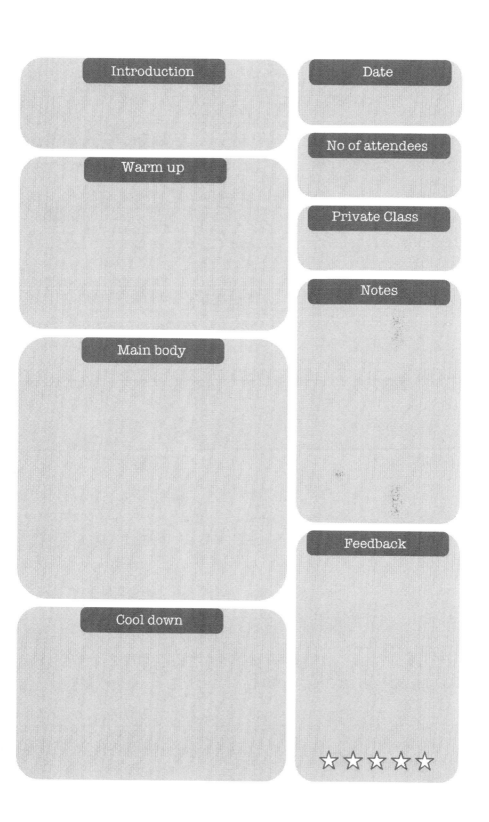

Introduction

Date

No of attendees

Private Class

Warm up

Notes

Main body

Feedback

Cool down

☆☆☆☆☆

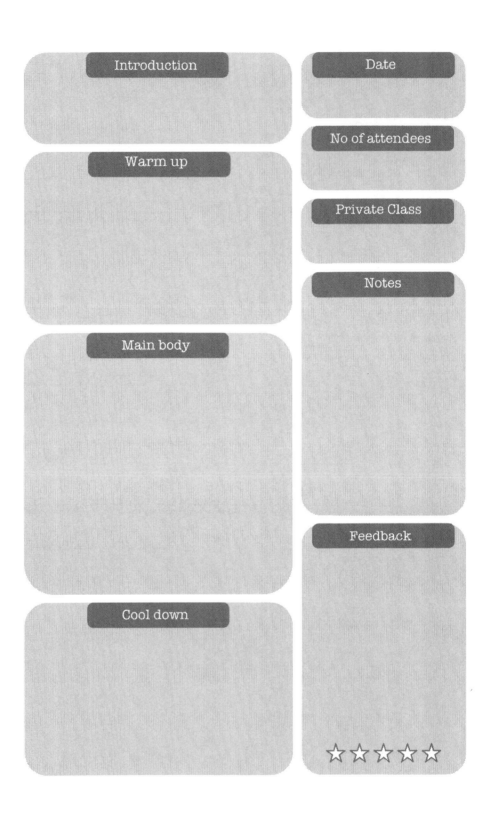

**Introduction**

**Date**

**Warm up**

**No of attendees**

**Private Class**

**Notes**

**Main body**

**Feedback**

**Cool down**

☆☆☆☆☆

## Introduction

## Date

## Warm up

## No of attendees

## Private Class

## Notes

## Main body

## Feedback

## Cool down

☆ ☆ ☆ ☆ ☆

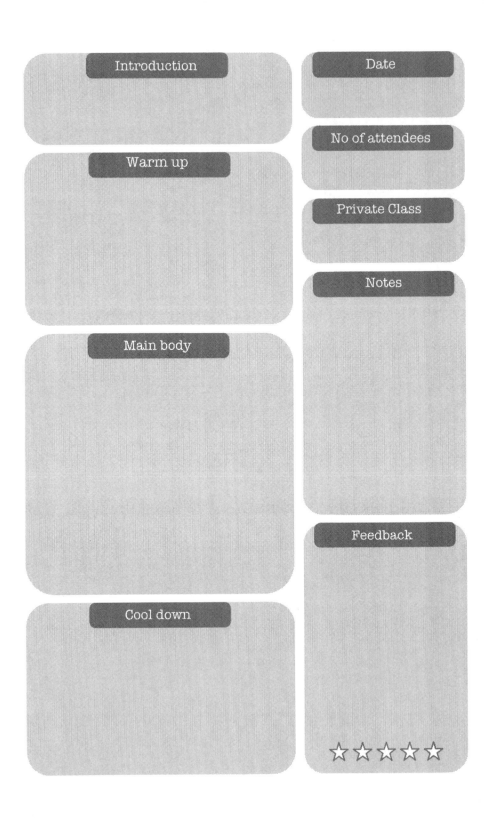

Introduction

Date

Warm up

No of attendees

Private Class

Main body

Notes

Feedback

Cool down

☆☆☆☆☆

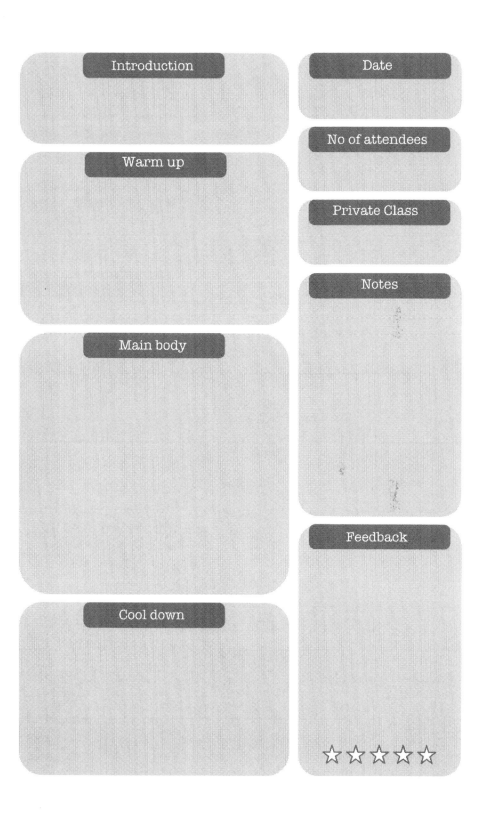

Introduction

Date

Warm up

No of attendees

Private Class

Main body

Notes

Cool down

Feedback

☆☆☆☆☆

## Introduction

## Warm up

## Main body

## Cool down

## Date

## No of attendees

## Private Class

## Notes

## Feedback

☆☆☆☆☆

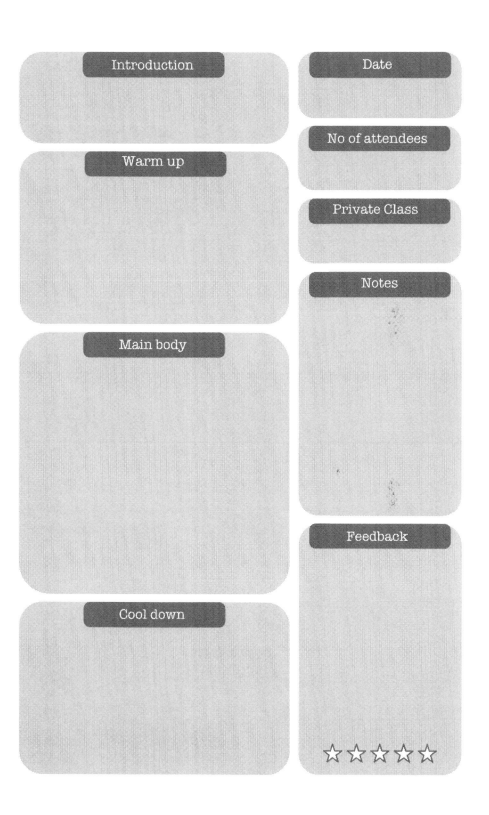

## Introduction

## Date

## Warm up

## No of attendees

## Private Class

## Main body

## Notes

## Feedback

## Cool down

☆ ☆ ☆ ☆ ☆

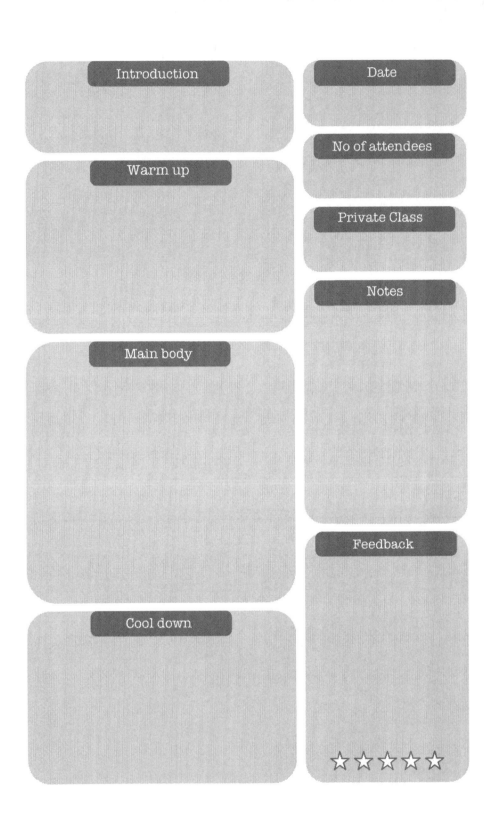

Introduction

Date

Warm up

No of attendees

Private Class

Main body

Notes

Feedback

Cool down

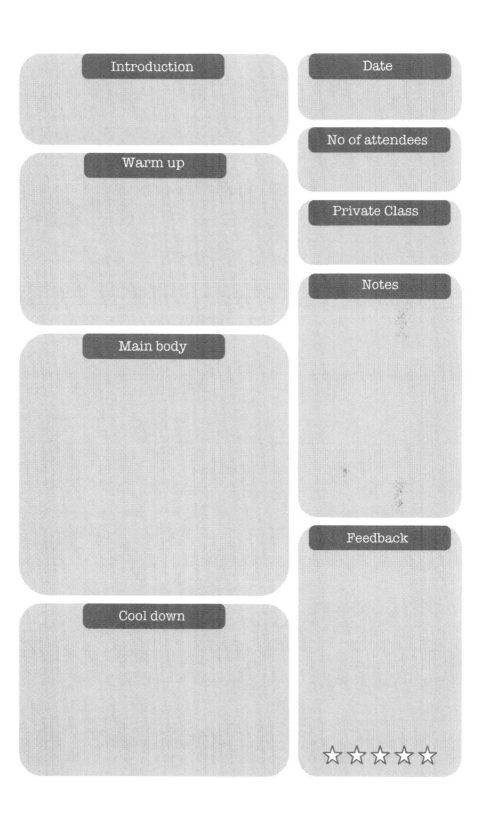

Introduction

Date

No of attendees

Private Class

Warm up

Notes

Main body

Feedback

Cool down

☆☆☆☆☆

## Introduction

## Date

## No of attendees

## Warm up

## Private Class

## Notes

## Main body

## Cool down

## Feedback

☆☆☆☆☆

## Introduction

## Warm up

## Main body

## Cool down

## Date

## No of attendees

## Private Class

## Notes

## Feedback

☆☆☆☆☆

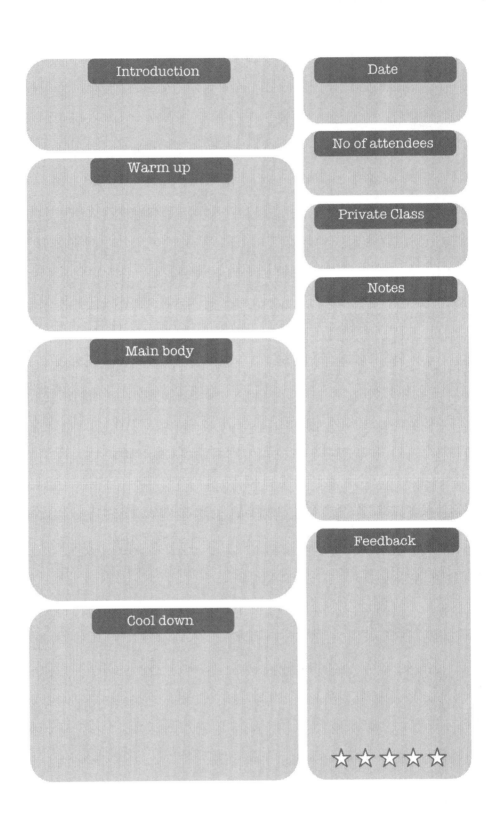

Introduction

Date

Warm up

No of attendees

Private Class

Main body

Notes

Feedback

Cool down

★ ★ ★ ★ ★

## Introduction

## Warm up

## Main body

## Cool down

## Date

## No of attendees

## Private Class

## Notes

## Feedback

☆☆☆☆☆

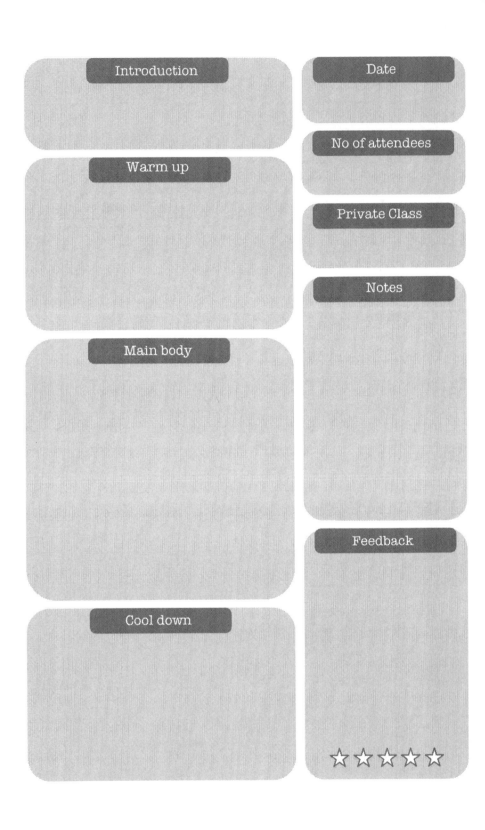

Introduction

Date

Warm up

No of attendees

Private Class

Main body

Notes

Feedback

Cool down

## Introduction

## Warm up

## Main body

## Cool down

## Date

## No of attendees

## Private Class

## Notes

## Feedback

☆☆☆☆☆

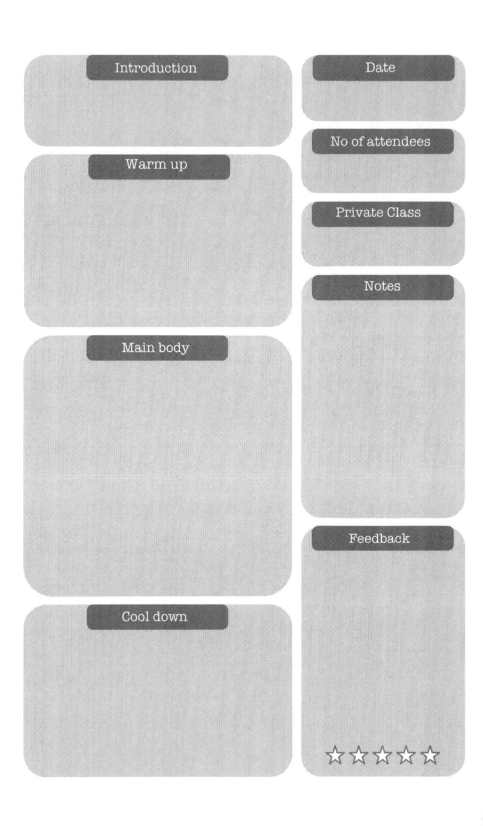

Introduction

Date

Warm up

No of attendees

Private Class

Main body

Notes

Feedback

Cool down

☆☆☆☆☆

## Introduction

## Date

## No of attendees

## Warm up

## Private Class

## Notes

## Main body

## Feedback

## Cool down

☆☆☆☆☆

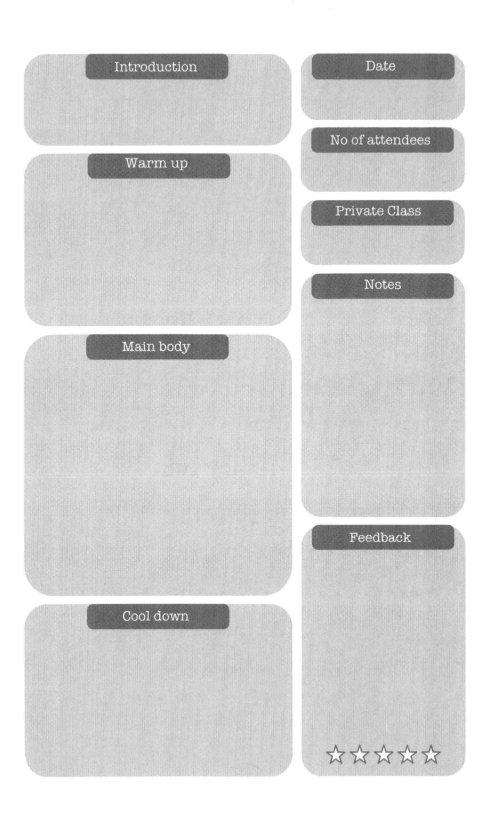

Introduction

Date

Warm up

No of attendees

Private Class

Main body

Notes

Feedback

Cool down

☆☆☆☆☆

**Introduction**

**Date**

**Warm up**

**No of attendees**

**Private Class**

**Notes**

**Main body**

**Feedback**

**Cool down**

☆☆☆☆☆

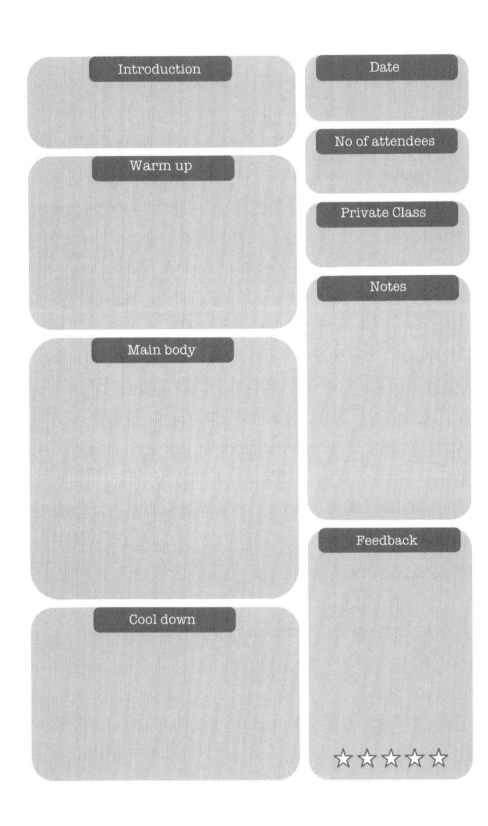

Introduction

Date

Warm up

No of attendees

Private Class

Main body

Notes

Feedback

Cool down

☆☆☆☆☆

## Introduction

## Date

## Warm up

## No of attendees

## Private Class

## Notes

## Main body

## Feedback

## Cool down

☆☆☆☆☆

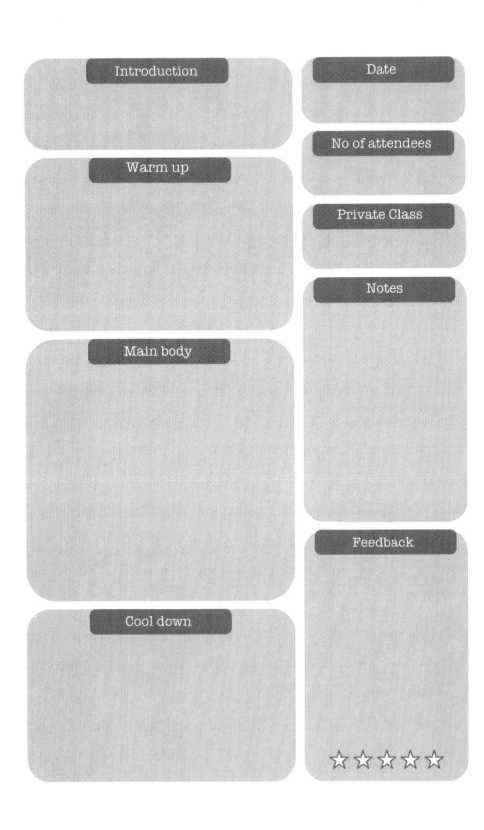

Introduction

Date

Warm up

No of attendees

Private Class

Main body

Notes

Feedback

Cool down

## Introduction

## Warm up

## Main body

## Cool down

## Date

## No of attendees

## Private Class

## Notes

## Feedback

☆☆☆☆☆

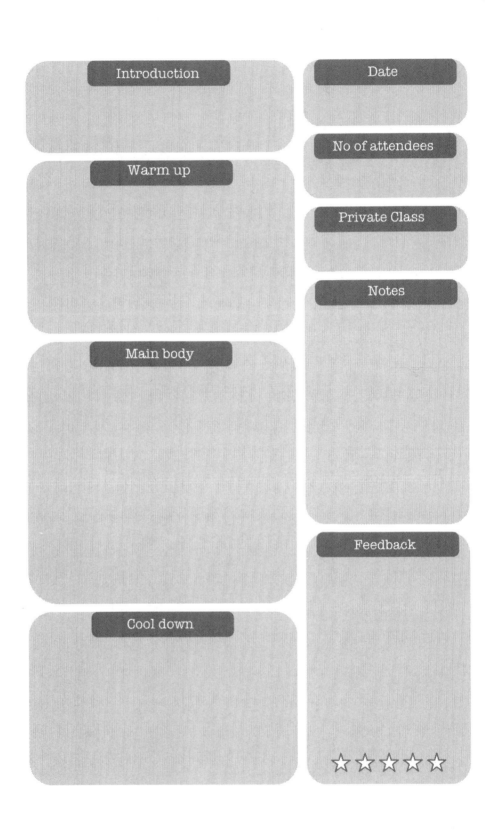

Introduction

Date

Warm up

No of attendees

Private Class

Main body

Notes

Feedback

Cool down

## Introduction

## Warm up

## Main body

## Cool down

## Date

## No of attendees

## Private Class

## Notes

## Feedback

☆☆☆☆☆

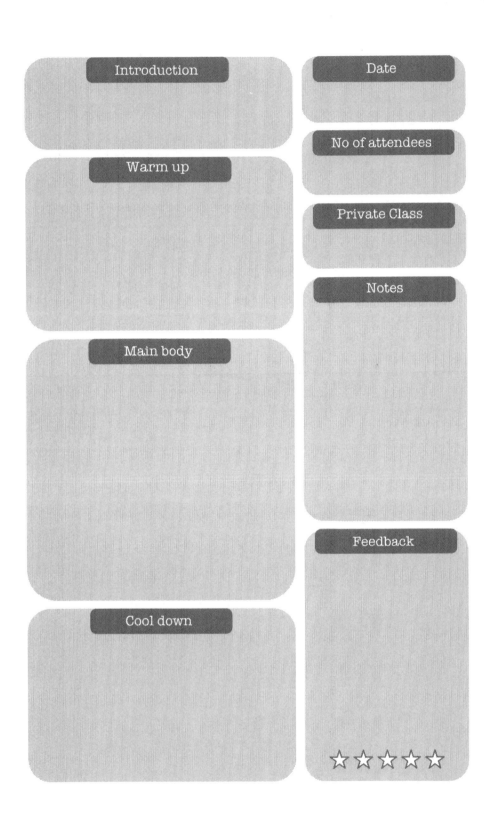

Introduction

Date

Warm up

No of attendees

Private Class

Main body

Notes

Feedback

Cool down

☆☆☆☆☆

## Introduction

## Date

## Warm up

## No of attendees

## Private Class

## Notes

## Main body

## Feedback

## Cool down

☆☆☆☆☆

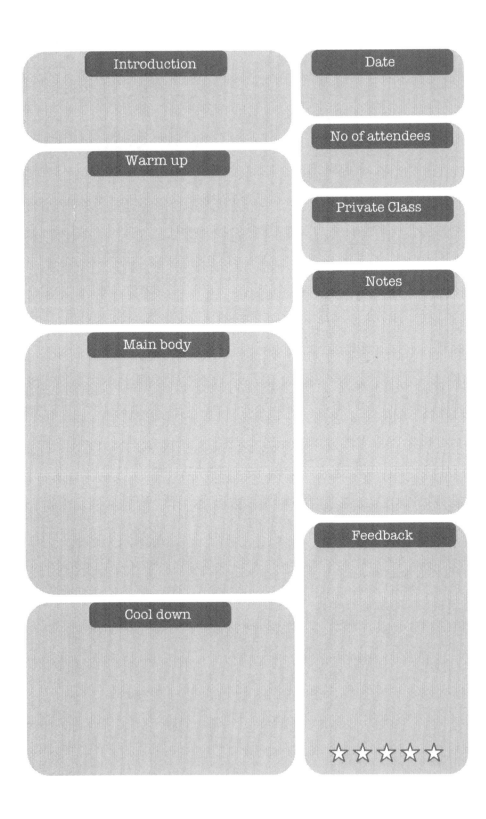

Introduction

Date

Warm up

No of attendees

Private Class

Main body

Notes

Feedback

Cool down

☆☆☆☆☆

## Introduction

## Date

## Warm up

## No of attendees

## Private Class

## Main body

## Notes

## Cool down

## Feedback

☆ ☆ ☆ ☆ ☆

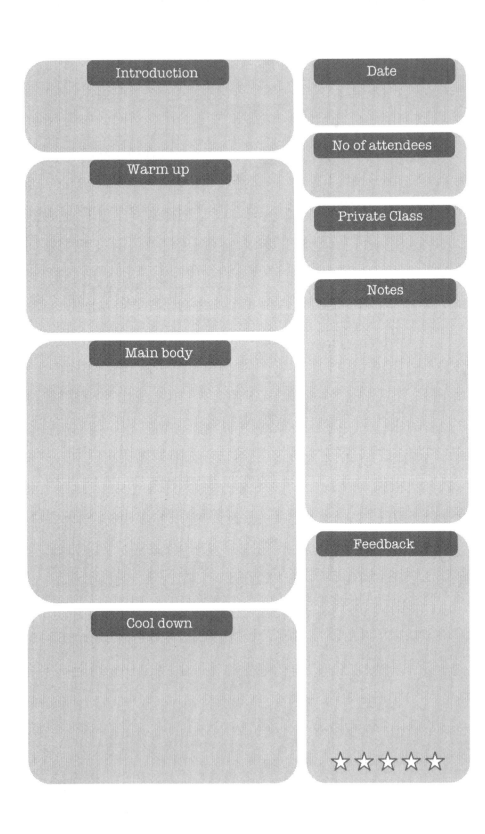

Introduction

Date

Warm up

No of attendees

Private Class

Main body

Notes

Feedback

Cool down

☆☆☆☆☆

## Introduction

## Warm up

## Main body

## Cool down

## Date

## No of attendees

## Private Class

## Notes

## Feedback

☆☆☆☆☆

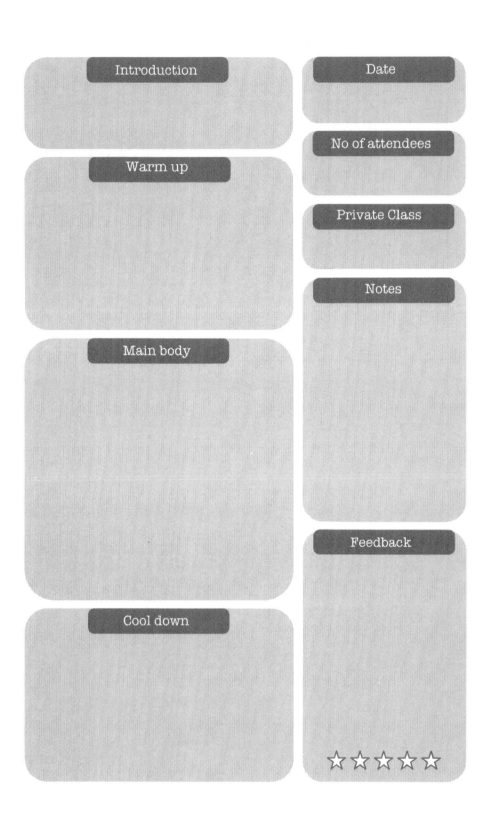

Introduction

Date

Warm up

No of attendees

Private Class

Main body

Notes

Cool down

Feedback

☆☆☆☆☆

## Introduction

## Date

## Warm up

## No of attendees

## Private Class

## Main body

## Notes

## Cool down

## Feedback

☆☆☆☆☆

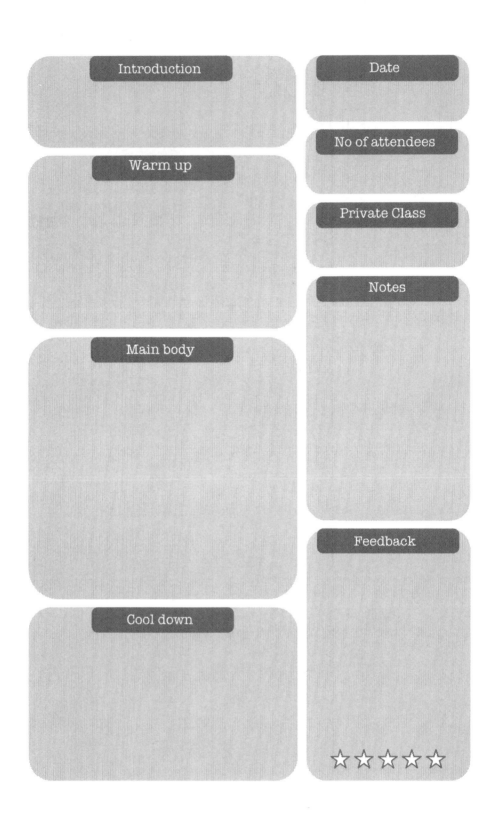

Introduction

Date

Warm up

No of attendees

Private Class

Main body

Notes

Cool down

Feedback

☆☆☆☆☆

## Introduction

## Warm up

## Main body

## Cool down

## Date

## No of attendees

## Private Class

## Notes

## Feedback

☆☆☆☆☆

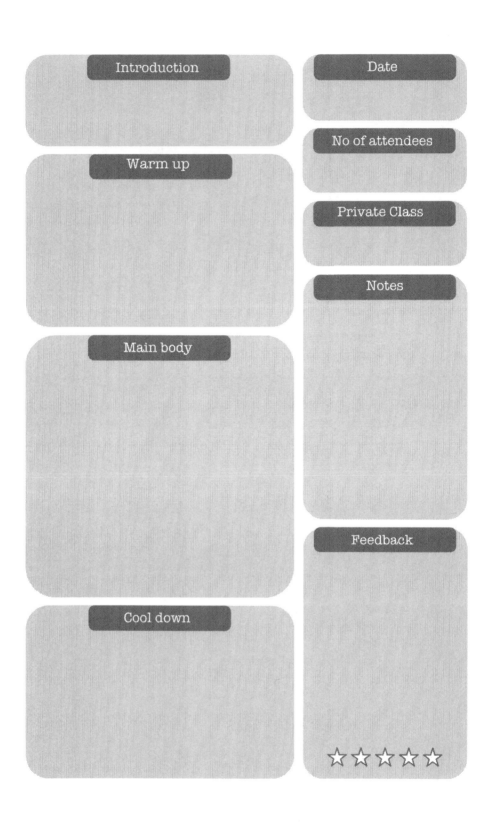

## Introduction

## Date

## Warm up

## No of attendees

## Private Class

## Notes

## Main body

## Feedback

## Cool down

☆☆☆☆☆

## Introduction

## Warm up

## Main body

## Cool down

## Date

## No of attendees

## Private Class

## Notes

## Feedback

☆ ☆ ☆ ☆ ☆

## Introduction

## Date

## Warm up

## No of attendees

## Private Class

## Main body

## Notes

## Feedback

## Cool down

☆☆☆☆☆

## Introduction

## Date

## Warm up

## No of attendees

## Private Class

## Main body

## Notes

## Feedback

## Cool down

☆☆☆☆☆

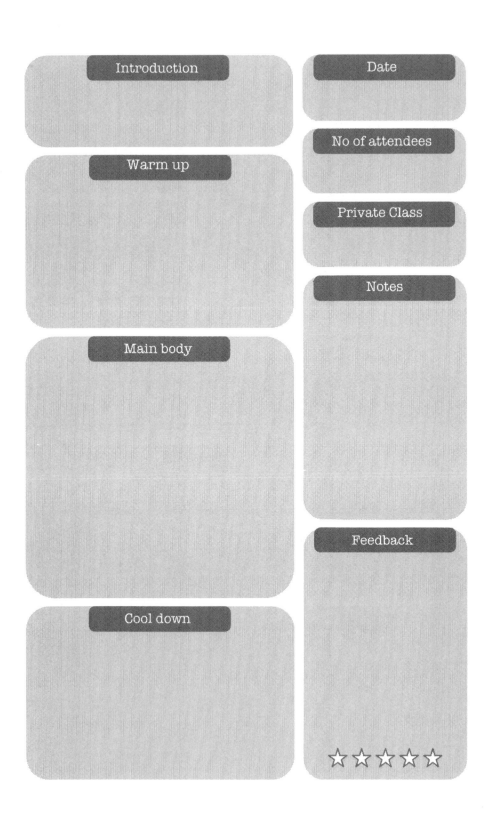

Introduction

Date

Warm up

No of attendees

Private Class

Main body

Notes

Feedback

Cool down

## Introduction

## Date

## Warm up

## No of attendees

## Private Class

## Notes

## Main body

## Feedback

## Cool down

☆☆☆☆☆

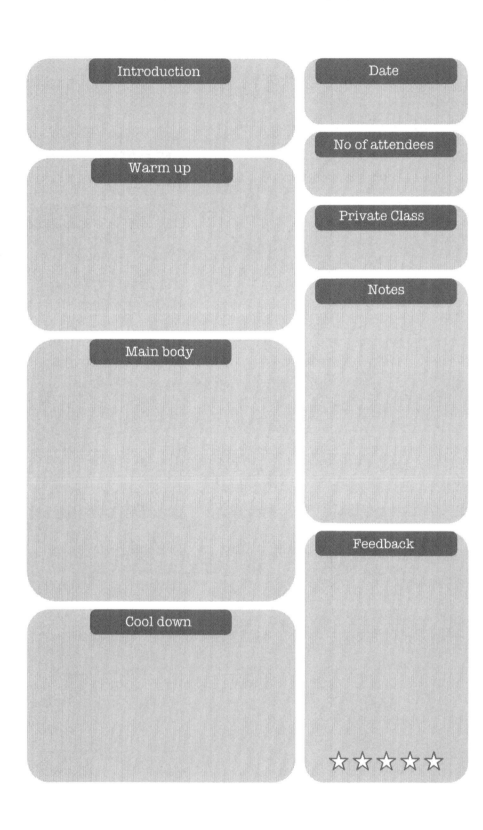

Introduction

Date

Warm up

No of attendees

Private Class

Main body

Notes

Feedback

Cool down

☆☆☆☆☆

## Introduction

## Date

## Warm up

## No of attendees

## Private Class

## Notes

## Main body

## Feedback

## Cool down

☆☆☆☆☆

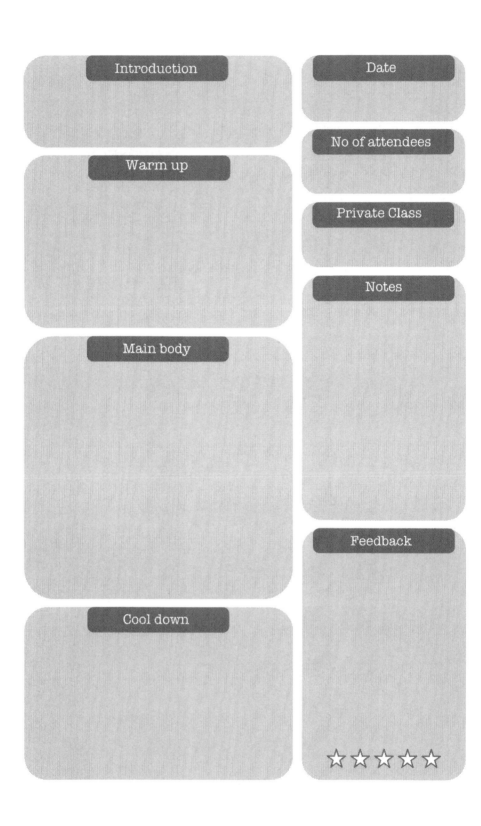

Introduction

Date

Warm up

No of attendees

Private Class

Main body

Notes

Feedback

Cool down

☆☆☆☆☆

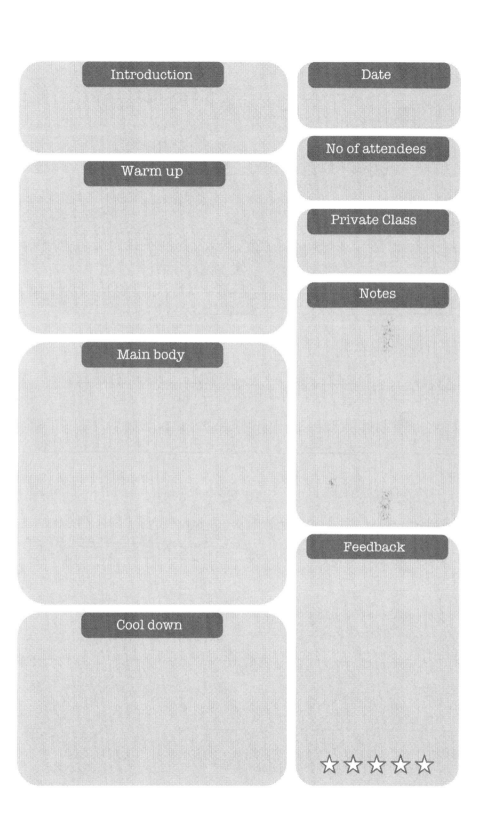

Introduction

Date

No of attendees

Warm up

Private Class

Notes

Main body

Feedback

Cool down

☆☆☆☆☆

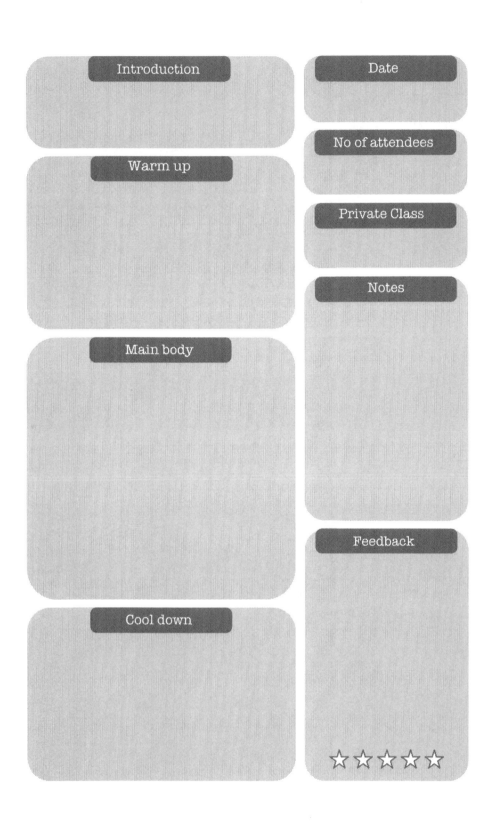

Introduction

Date

Warm up

No of attendees

Private Class

Main body

Notes

Cool down

Feedback

☆☆☆☆☆

## Introduction

## Warm up

## Main body

## Cool down

## Date

## No of attendees

## Private Class

## Notes

## Feedback

☆ ☆ ☆ ☆ ☆

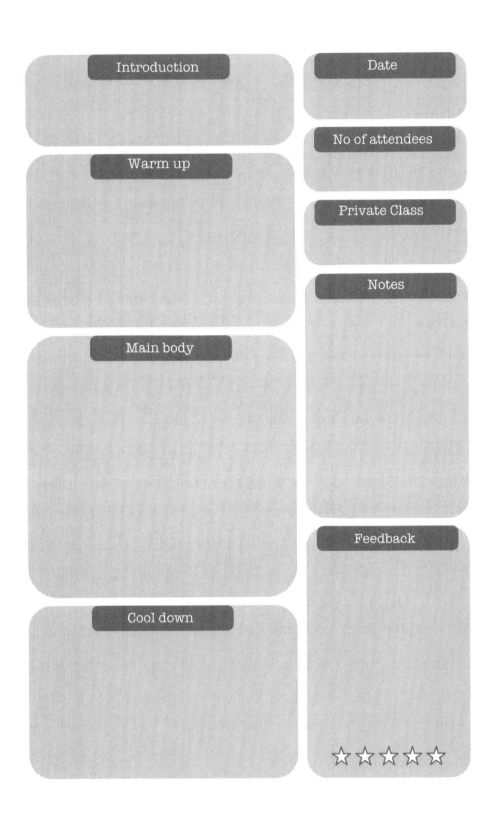

Introduction

Date

Warm up

No of attendees

Private Class

Main body

Notes

Feedback

Cool down

☆☆☆☆☆

## Introduction

## Date

## Warm up

## No of attendees

## Private Class

## Notes

## Main body

## Feedback

## Cool down

☆ ☆ ☆ ☆ ☆

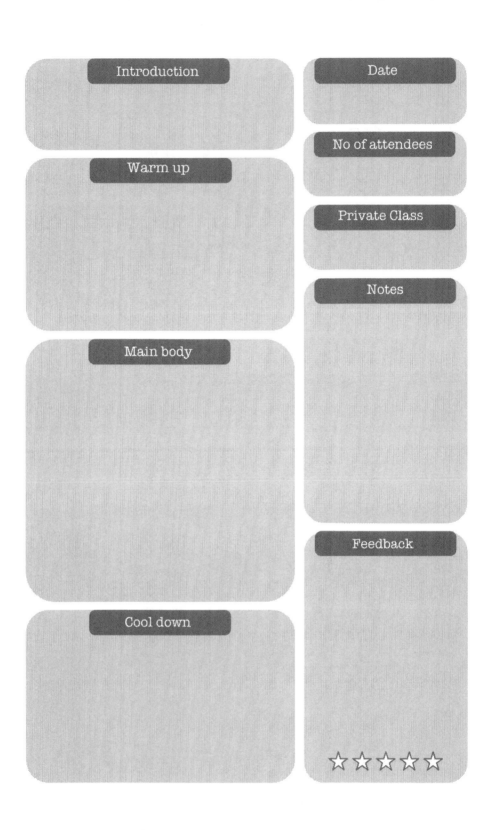

Introduction

Date

Warm up

No of attendees

Private Class

Notes

Main body

Feedback

Cool down

☆☆☆☆☆

## Introduction

## Warm up

## Main body

## Cool down

## Date

## No of attendees

## Private Class

## Notes

## Feedback

☆☆☆☆☆

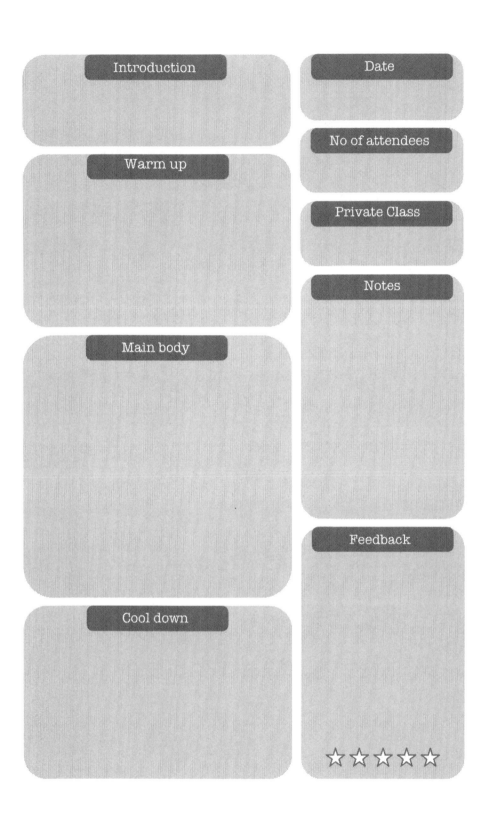

Introduction

Date

Warm up

No of attendees

Private Class

Main body

Notes

Feedback

Cool down

★★★★★

## Introduction

## Warm up

## Main body

## Cool down

## Date

## No of attendees

## Private Class

## Notes

## Feedback

☆ ☆ ☆ ☆ ☆

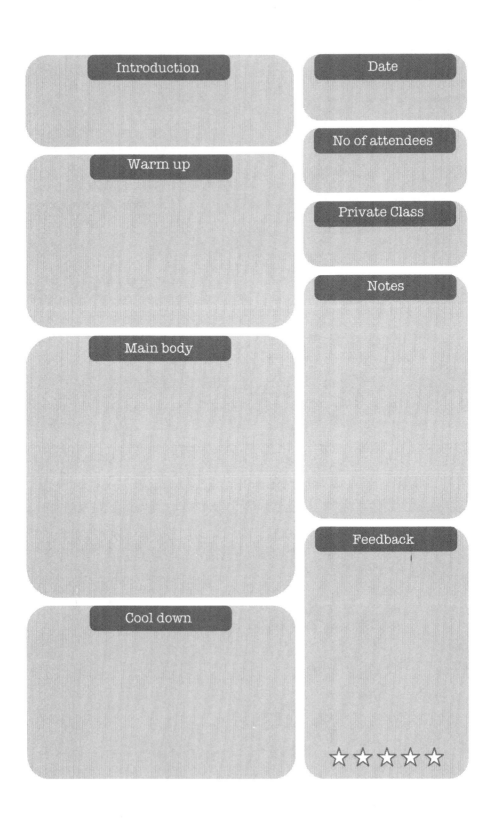

Introduction

Date

Warm up

No of attendees

Private Class

Main body

Notes

Feedback

Cool down

☆☆☆☆☆

## Introduction

## Date

## Warm up

## No of attendees

## Private Class

## Notes

## Main body

## Feedback

## Cool down

☆ ☆ ☆ ☆ ☆

Introduction

Date

Warm up

No of attendees

Private Class

Main body

Notes

Feedback

Cool down

☆ ☆ ☆ ☆ ☆

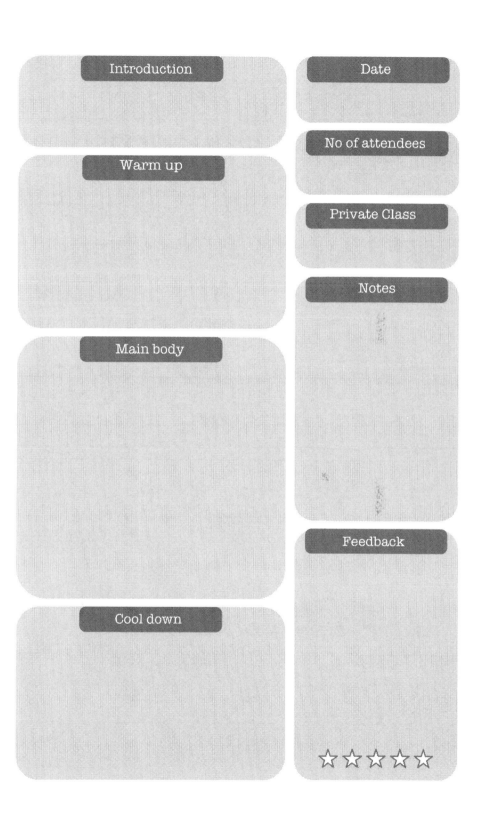

Introduction

Date

Warm up

No of attendees

Private Class

Main body

Notes

Feedback

Cool down

☆ ☆ ☆ ☆ ☆

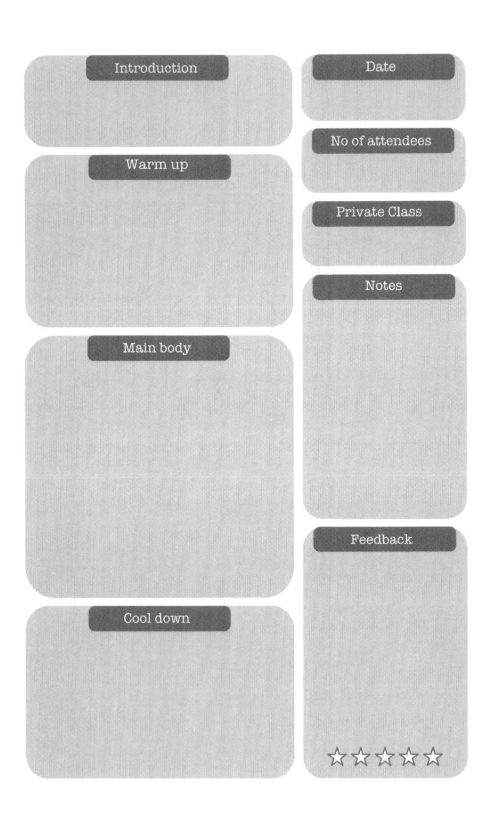

Introduction

Date

Warm up

No of attendees

Private Class

Main body

Notes

Feedback

Cool down

☆☆☆☆☆

## Introduction

## Date

## Warm up

## No of attendees

## Private Class

## Main body

## Notes

## Cool down

## Feedback

☆ ☆ ☆ ☆ ☆

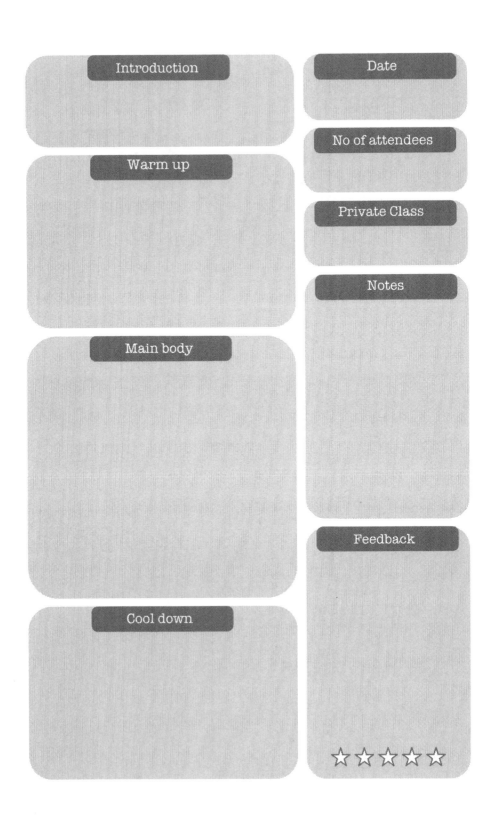

Introduction

Date

No of attendees

Private Class

Warm up

Notes

Main body

Feedback

Cool down

☆☆☆☆☆

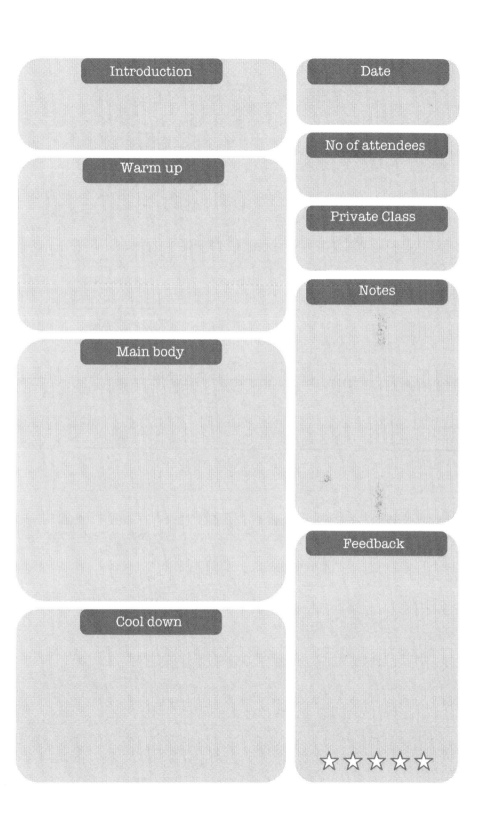

Introduction

Date

Warm up

No of attendees

Private Class

Main body

Notes

Cool down

Feedback

☆☆☆☆☆

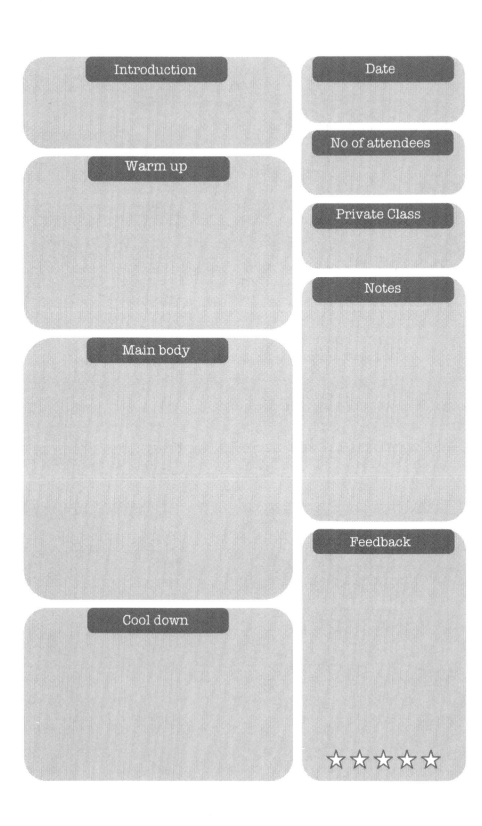

Introduction

Date

Warm up

No of attendees

Private Class

Main body

Notes

Feedback

Cool down

☆☆☆☆☆

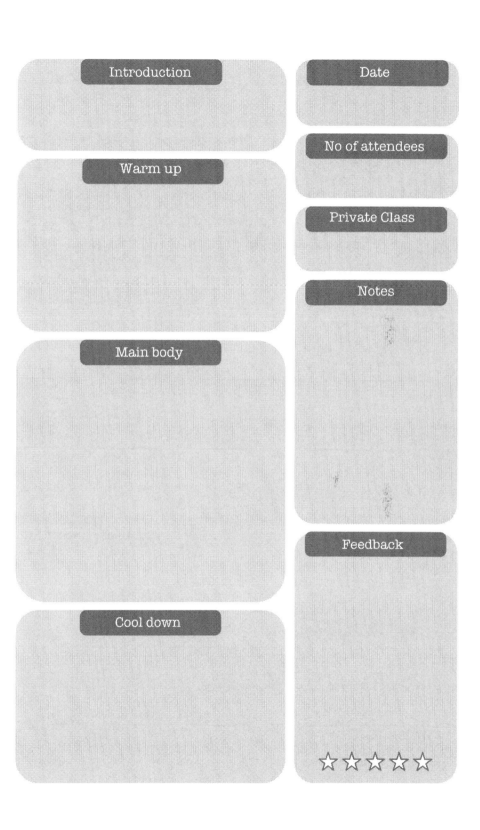

Introduction

Date

Warm up

No of attendees

Private Class

Main body

Notes

Feedback

Cool down

☆☆☆☆☆

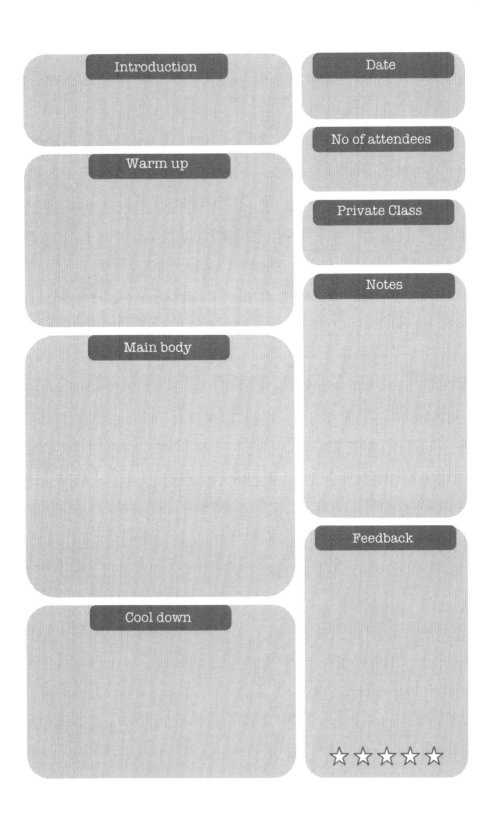

**Introduction**

**Date**

**Warm up**

**No of attendees**

**Private Class**

**Notes**

**Main body**

**Feedback**

**Cool down**

☆☆☆☆☆

## Introduction

## Date

## Warm up

## No of attendees

## Private Class

## Notes

## Main body

## Cool down

## Feedback

☆☆☆☆☆

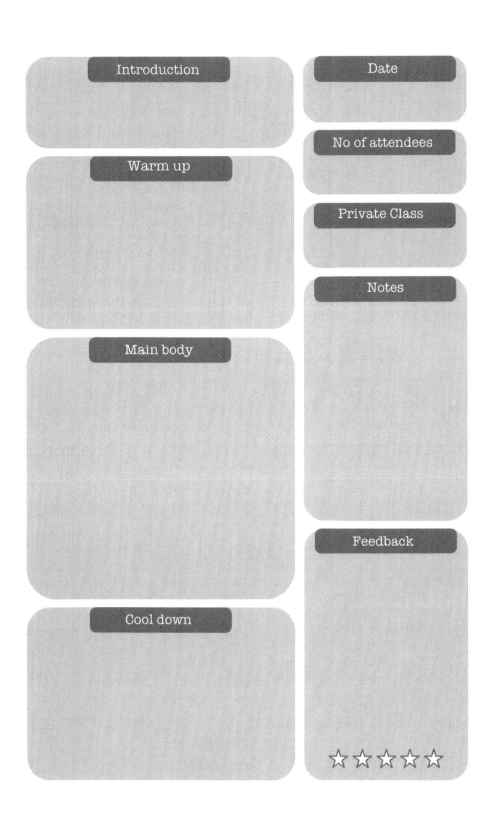

Introduction

Date

Warm up

No of attendees

Private Class

Main body

Notes

Cool down

Feedback

☆☆☆☆☆

## Introduction

## Date

## No of attendees

## Warm up

## Private Class

## Notes

## Main body

## Feedback

## Cool down

☆ ☆ ☆ ☆ ☆

Notes

61007860R00062

Made in the USA
Middletown, DE
17 August 2019